THE ULTIMATE HASHIMOTO PALEO COOKBOOK

Delicious Hashimoto's Thyroiditis Diet Recipes & Food List for Thyroid Health with 2-Week Meal Plan.

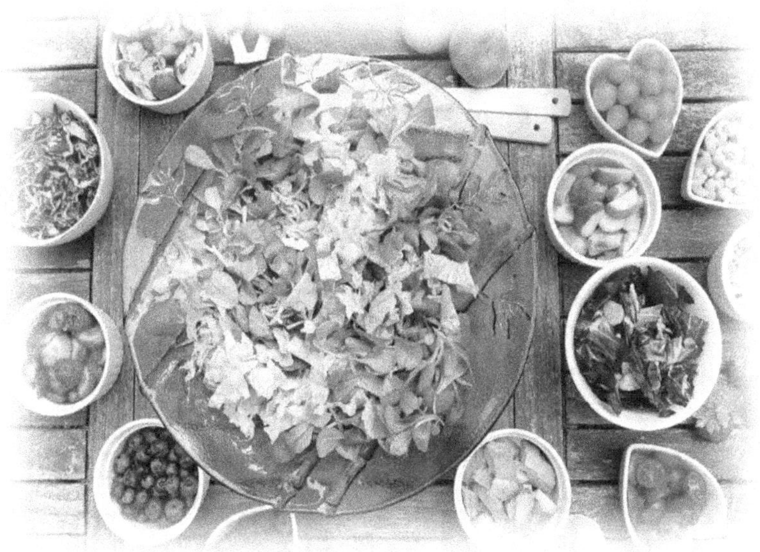

CHRISTIANA WHITE.

GAIN ACCESS TO MORE BOOKS

TABLE OF CONTENTS.

INTRODUCTION

Enter a world where overcoming Hashimoto's thyroiditis becomes a delicious, healing gastronomic adventure. Introducing Sarah: formerly veiled in exhaustion, she has been reenergized by the Hashimoto Paleo Cookbook. Her experience offers insight into the transformational potential of this recipe book.

Every recipe in these pages is a flavorful mosaic designed to energize and nourish. This cookbook is a lifeline for a community dealing with the difficulties of Hashimoto's disease, more than just a compilation of recipes. It's a pledge that if we work together, we can make every meal a celebration of health.

Why is this book important? Because it not only reveals the key to treating Hashimoto's disease but also the delight of relishing every mouthful while pursuing well-being. It's a supportive network, a customized guide, and evidence of the vibrancy that arises when intention and sustenance come together.

As a thank you, special recipes entice with the promise of a magnificent path toward a happier, healthier you. Join the group of people who have discovered a lifestyle, not just a diet, with the Hashimoto Paleo Cookbook, where deliciousness and healing come together in harmony. Embrace a life where each meal is an opportunity to become the best version of yourself.

CHAPTER 1

Understanding Hashimoto's

This chapter delves into the complexities of an autoimmune disease, examining its effects on the thyroid gland and the larger picture of our health. With a brief investigation, we hope to arm you with knowledge that establishes the foundation for wise dietary decisions and a well-coordinated strategy for managing your Hashimoto's.

Hashimoto's Thyroiditis Overview

Hypothyroidism is the outcome of Hashimoto's thyroiditis, an inflammatory illness that damages the thyroid gland and induces persistent inflammation. The thyroid gland produces inadequate thyroid hormone, which causes hypothyroidism. Thyroid hormones control the body's growth, development, and metabolism. About 5% of people in the US suffer from hypothyroidism due to Hashimoto's thyroiditis, which is most frequent in women and older adults.

Although the precise origin of Hashimoto's thyroiditis is unknown, hormonal, environmental, and genetic variables are thought to play a role.

Some of the frequent symptoms of Hashimoto's thyroiditis include fatigue, weight gain, cold intolerance, dry skin, hair loss, constipation, depression, and monthly abnormalities.Hashimoto's thyroiditis is diagnosed by testing the levels of thyroid hormones and thyroid antibodies in the blood.

Synthetic thyroid hormone replacement treatment is used to treat Hashimoto's thyroiditis. This improves symptoms and returns thyroid hormone levels to normal.Hashimoto's thyroiditis is a chronic illness that needs to be regularly monitored and treated with medication adjustments.

Effect on the Gland of Thyroid

The thyroid gland is a butterfly-shaped structure found near the base of the neck, which generates two primary hormones: thyroxine (T4) and triiodothyronine (T3).The body's ability to produce energy, regulate temperature, heart rate, blood pressure, growth, and development all depend on these hormones.

In the brain, the pituitary gland and the hypothalamus work together to regulate the production and secretion of thyroid hormones, creating a feedback loop.

The pituitary gland releases thyroid-stimulating hormone (TSH) in response to the release of thyrotropin-releasing hormone (TRH) from the hypothalamus. TSH then stimulates the thyroid gland to create T4 and T3.

The hypothalamus and pituitary gland, respectively, lower their secretions of TRH and TSH to preserve equilibrium when T4 and T3 levels are sufficient. When the immune system unintentionally targets the thyroid gland, it causes antibodies that disrupt the gland's structure and function, leading to Hashimoto's thyroiditis.

This causes the thyroid tissue to gradually deteriorate, which lowers the thyroid's hormone production. The brain and pituitary gland secrete more TRH and TSH, respectively, in response to a reduction in T4 and T3, which stimulates the thyroid gland to create additional hormones.

The characteristic of hypothyroidism, a continuous elevation of TSH and low levels of T4 and T3, results from the thyroid gland's inability to meet the increased demand. Nodules, cysts, or goiters—abnormal enlargements of the thyroid gland that can alter its function and appearance—can also develop as a result of long-term inflammation and damage to the gland.

The Diet's Function in Symptom Management

The management of Hashimoto's thyroiditis symptoms is significantly influenced by diet, as certain foods can exacerbate or cause inflammation, autoimmune, and thyroid dysfunction, while other foods can promote healing and enhance overall well-being.

The following are a few dietary variables that may influence Hashimoto's thyroiditis:

• **Iodine**: The production of thyroid hormones requires the trace mineral iodine. On the other hand, an excess or deficiency of iodine can induce or worsen Hashimoto's thyroiditis by interfering with thyroid function.

As a result, it's critical to get enough iodine from diet and supplements—not too much, though. The recommended dietary allowance (RDA) for iodine is 150 mcg per day for adults. Seaweed, seafood, dairy products, eggs, and iodized salt are a few foods high in iodine.

• **Gluten**: Barley, rye, wheat, and certain other cereals contain the protein gluten. Because gluten can cross-react with thyroid tissue and promote the formation of thyroid antibodies, it can cause an immunological response in certain individuals with Hashimoto's thyroiditis.

Intestinal permeability, also known as leaky gut, is a disorder in which the gut lining is injured and permits germs, toxins, and undigested food particles to enter the bloodstream, leading to inflammation and autoimmune. Gluten can also exacerbate this disease.

Therefore, for some individuals with Hashimoto's thyroiditis, removing gluten from the diet may help lower symptoms and antibody levels.

• **Dairy**: Due to the presence of casein, a protein that can react with thyroid tissue and raise the generation of thyroid antibodies, dairy products may also cause an immunological reaction in certain Hashimoto's thyroiditis patients.

Dairy products can also trigger inflammation and leaky gut in certain people who are sensitive or intolerant to lactose, the sugar contained in milk. Therefore, in some cases of Hashimoto's thyroiditis, removing dairy from the diet can help lower antibody levels and symptoms.

• **Soy**: Because soy products contain isoflavones, which are plant components that can operate in the body as weak estrogen substitutes, they may interfere with the thyroid gland's ability to secrete thyroid hormone and the body's ability to absorb medicine.

In some cases of Hashimoto's thyroiditis, soy products can also provoke an immunological response because they contain lectins, which are proteins that attach to gut cells and induce inflammation and leaky gut.

For this reason, in certain cases of Hashimoto's thyroiditis, reducing or eliminating soy products can enhance the efficacy of thyroid hormone therapy and thyroid function.

• **Goitrogens**: These compounds have the ability to prevent the thyroid gland from absorbing iodine and to obstruct the thyroid gland's ability to produce thyroid hormones. Cruciferous vegetables (broccoli, cabbage, cauliflower, kale, and Brussels sprouts), millet, cassava, peanuts, and strawberries are a few foods that contain goitrogens.

Nonetheless, goitrogens often have moderate effects, which can be mitigated by boiling or fermenting these foods. Therefore, unless they have a severe iodine deficit or consume high amounts of goitrogens, most persons with Hashimoto's thyroiditis are unlikely to experience issues with consuming modest amounts of these foods as part of a balanced diet.

• **Selenium**: A trace mineral, selenium helps transform T4 into T3, the more potent type of thyroid hormone. Additionally, the anti-inflammatory and antioxidant qualities of selenium can lessen the synthesis of thyroid antibodies and shield the thyroid gland from oxidative damage.

As a result, for certain individuals with Hashimoto's thyroiditis, getting enough selenium from food or supplements can help regulate the thyroid and lessen symptoms and antibody levels.

Adults should consume 55 mg of selenium daily3.Selenium-rich foods include eggs, mushrooms, pork, poultry, shellfish, Brazil nuts, and fowl.

• **Zinc**: Another trace mineral, zinc has a role in the transformation of T4 into T3, as well as in the hypothalamus-pituitary-thyroid axis regulation that governs thyroid hormone release. In addition to its anti-inflammatory and antioxidant qualities, zinc can help lower the generation of thyroid antibodies and shield the thyroid gland from oxidative damage.

Thus, for certain individuals with Hashimoto's thyroiditis, obtaining sufficient zinc from food or supplements will help regulate the thyroid and lessen symptoms and antibody levels.

The recommended daily allowance (RDA) for zinc is 8 mg for women and 11 mg for men3.Chickpeas, cashews, pumpkin seeds, lamb, oysters, and lamb are a few foods high in zinc.

Based on the concepts of the Paleo diet, the Hashimoto Paleo Diet is a dietary strategy tailored to the needs of individuals with Hashimoto's thyroiditis. All forms of gluten, dairy, soy, and processed foods are excluded from the Hashimoto Paleo Diet, along with the majority of grains, legumes, and nightshade vegetables (including tomatoes, potatoes, peppers, and eggplants), which may cause allergies or inflammation in certain individuals.

Nutrient-dense foods, such as organic or grass-fed meats, wild-caught fish, organ meats, bone broth, eggs, nuts, seeds, fruits, and vegetables—especially those high in zinc, iodine, and selenium—are the mainstay of the Hashimoto Paleo diet.

The Hashimoto Paleo Diet also promotes the use of herbs and spices that have anti-inflammatory and antioxidant properties, including as turmeric, ginger, garlic, and cinnamon, as well as healthy fats like avocado, coconut oil, olive oil, and ghee.

In some cases, the Hashimoto Paleo Diet can help relieve the symptoms of Hashimoto's thyroiditis by lowering inflammation, healing leaky gut, boosting immunity, and enhancing thyroid function.

But it's crucial to remember that there are individual differences and preferences to consider, and that the Hashimoto Paleo Diet is not a one-size-fits-all approach. Depending on their individual tolerance and reaction, some people might benefit from further eliminating or reintroducing particular foods.

Certain individuals may also require dietary supplements of specific nutrients, including vitamin B12, iron, or D, based on their blood test results and symptoms. A trained medical expert should supervise the Hashimoto Paleo Diet.

They may evaluate thyroid function, change medication dosages, and offer personalized direction and support. Although there is no known treatment for Hashimoto's thyroiditis, some people may find that their quality of life is improved and their disease is better managed with the Hashimoto Paleo Diet.

CHAPTER 2

Breakfast Recipes

Keto Breakfast Burger with Avocado Buns

(2 serves, 15 minutes preparation)

Ingredients:

- 2 ground beef patties (4 ounces each)
- Two avocados, halved and pitted
- Four pieces of bacon
- Two fried eggs.
- 1 tablespoon mayonnaise.
- One teaspoon Dijon mustard
- Lettuce leaves
- Sliced tomatoes (optional)

Method:

- Season the ground beef with salt and pepper. Form into patties and cook to your preferred doneness.
- While the beef cooks, sauté the bacon strips until crispy.
- Cook eggs till easy or medium.
- Combine avocado halves, lemon juice, and salt to make "buns."

- Spread mayonnaise and mustard over avocado buns. Add lettuce, ground beef patty, bacon, fried egg, and tomato (optional).

Paleo Freezer Breakfast Burritos.

(5 serves, 20 minutes preparation, 15 minutes cooking)

Ingredients:

- 5 big, scrambled eggs
- 1/2 cup of diced onion.
- 1/2 cup of chopped bell pepper.
- 1/4 cup of chopped mushrooms.
- 1/4 cup cooked bacon or sausage (optional).
- One cup of spinach.
- Five huge lettuce leaves.
- One avocado, sliced

Method:

- In a skillet, heat the olive oil and cook the onion, bell pepper, and mushrooms until tender. Add the sausage or bacon and heat until browned.
- Scramble the eggs, then stir in the spinach until wilted.

- Make burritos by putting out lettuce leaves and stacking with scrambled eggs, sausage/bacon, and avocado slices. Roll up tightly and wrap with parchment paper. Freeze for up to three months.
- Thaw overnight in the refrigerator or microwave for 1-2 minutes until heated through.

Paleo Red Flannel Hash.

(4 serves, 15 minutes preparation, 20 minutes cooking)

Ingredients:

- Two medium sweet potatoes, cubed.
- 1/2 cup of diced onion.
- 1/2 cup of diced red bell pepper.
- 1/4 cup chopped bacon or ham.
- 2 tablespoons olive oil.
- Add salt and pepper to taste.

Method:

- In a pan, heat olive oil over medium heat. heat. Cook for about 5 minutes, or until the onion and bell pepper soften.
- Add the diced sweet potatoes and simmer for another 10-15 minutes, stirring regularly, until soft and golden.

- Add ham or bacon and season with salt and pepper to taste. Serve with fried eggs, if preferred.

Keto Blueberry Muffins

(12 muffins, 15 minutes preparation, 20 minutes cooking)

Ingredients:

- One cup of almond flour.
- One-quarter cup coconut flour
- 1/2 teaspoon baking powder.
- 1/4 teaspoon baking soda.
- 1/4 teaspoon salt.
- 1/4 cup of melted grass-fed butter.
- Three big eggs.
- 1/4 cup honey or maple syrup.
- 1/4 cup of unsweetened almond milk.
- One-half cup blueberries

Method:

- Preheat the oven to 350°F (175° C). Line the muffin tray with paper liners.
- In a bowl, combine almond flour, coconut flour, baking powder, baking soda, and salt.

- In a separate bowl, whisk together the melted butter, eggs, maple syrup or honey, and almond milk.
- Mix together the wet and dry ingredients until just mixed. Fold in blueberries.
- Pour batter into muffin cups and bake for 15-20 minutes, or until a toothpick inserted in the center comes out clean. Let cool before serving.

Bacon & Egg Sweet Potato Pancake Breakfast Sandwich

(2 serves, 15 minutes preparation, 10 minutes cooking)

Ingredients:

- One medium sweet potato, shredded
- 1 egg
- One tablespoon of almond flour.
- 1/4 teaspoon cinnamon.
- A pinch of salt.
- Two pieces of bacon
- Two fried eggs.
- Two slices avocado (optional)

Method:

- In a bowl, combine the grated sweet potato, egg, almond flour, cinnamon, and salt. Mix until thoroughly mixed.
- Heat a frying pan over medium heat with olive oil. Pour the batter into two equal-sized circles and cook for 2-3 minutes on each side, or until golden brown.

Loaded Paleo Breakfast Hash.

(4 serves, 15 minutes preparation, 20 minutes cooking)

Ingredients:

- Two medium sweet potatoes, cubed.
- 1/2 cup of diced onion.
- 1/2 cup of chopped bell pepper.
- 1/4 cup of chopped mushrooms.
- 4 pieces of bacon, diced
- Four fried eggs.
- 1/4 cup crumbled goat cheese.
- 1/4 cup diced avocado.
- Fresh herbs (optional).

Method:

- In a pan, heat olive oil over medium heat.Cook for about 5 minutes, or until the onion, bell pepper, and mushrooms soften.
- Add the diced sweet potatoes and simmer for another 10-15 minutes, stirring regularly, until soft and golden.
- Stir in the chopped bacon and heat for another minute.
- Add fried eggs, goat cheese, avocado, and fresh herbs (optional).

Make-Ahead Breakfast Sandwich

(4 servings, 15 minutes preparation, 10 minutes cooking)

Ingredients:

- Four sausage or ground beef patties.
- Four fried eggs.
- 4 whole-wheat hamburger buns (or lettuce wraps for Paleo)
- One avocado, sliced
- Tomato slices (optional).
- Dijon mustard (Optional)

Method:

- Cook sausage or ground beef patties according to the package directions.
- Cook eggs till easy or medium.
- Make sandwiches by putting sausage/beef patties on buns and topping with fried eggs, avocado slices, and tomato (optional). Spread Dijon mustard on the bun's bottom or top, as desired.
- Wrap sandwiches tightly in plastic wrap and refrigerate for up to three days. Reheat in the microwave for 1-2 minutes until heated through.

Paleo Porridge with Caramelized Bananas

(2 serves, 10 minutes preparation, 15 minutes cooking)

Ingredients:

- 1 cup of chopped mixed nuts and seeds (almonds, walnuts, pumpkin seeds, sunflower seeds).
- 1/2 cup of unsweetened almond milk.
- One-quarter cup coconut milk
- 1/4 teaspoon cinnamon.
- A pinch of salt.
- One banana, sliced

- One tablespoon of coconut oil.

Method:

- In a saucepan, mix together the nuts and seeds, almond milk, coconut milk, cinnamon, and salt. Bring to a simmer, then cook for 5 minutes.
- Meanwhile, heat the coconut oil in a separate pan over medium heat. Cook the sliced banana until it is softened and caramelized.
- Top warm porridge with caramelized bananas and enjoy!

Zucchini Carrot Muffins

(12 muffins, 15 minutes preparation, 20 minutes cooking)

Ingredients:

- One cup shredded zucchini.
- One-half cup grated carrots
- One-quarter cup almond flour
- One-quarter cup coconut flour
- 1/4 teaspoon baking powder.
- 1/4 teaspoon baking soda.
- 1/4 teaspoon salt.
- 2 eggs

- 1/4 cup honey or maple syrup.

- 1/4 cup of unsweetened almond milk.

Method:

- Preheat the oven to 350°F (175° C). Line the muffin tray with paper liners.

- In a mixing dish, add grated zucchini, carrots, almond flour, coconut flour, baking powder, baking soda, and salt. Allow for 5 minutes to absorb moisture.

- In a separate bowl, whisk together the eggs, maple syrup or honey, and almond milk.

- Mix together the wet and dry ingredients until just mixed.

- Pour batter into muffin cups and bake for 15-20 minutes, or until a toothpick inserted in the center comes out clean. Let cool before serving.

Baked Almond Quinoa with Oatmeal

(4 servings, 15 minutes preparation, 25 minutes cooking)

Ingredients:

- 1/2 cup washed quinoa.
- One-half cup almond flour
- 1/4 cup rolled oats.
- 1/4 teaspoon baking powder.
- A pinch of salt.
- One cup unsweetened almond milk.
- 2 eggs
- 1/4 cup honey or maple syrup.
- 1/4 cup of chopped nuts (optional).

Method:

- Preheat the oven to 350°F (175°C). Grease a baking dish or individual ramekins. Line the dish with parchment paper to make cleanup easy.
- In a medium bowl, combine the quinoa, almond flour, rolled oats, baking powder, and salt.
- In a separate bowl, combine almond milk, eggs, and maple syrup/honey.

- Add the wet ingredients to the dry ingredients and mix until just mixed. Avoid overmixing because it can make the oatmeal gritty.

- Fold in the chopped nuts, if using. You can choose walnuts, almonds, pecans, or any other nut you like.

- Transfer the batter to the prepared baking dish or individual ramekins. Spread it evenly.

- A toothpick inserted in the center should come out clean after baking for 25 to 30 minutes, or until the cake is golden brown.

- Allow the oatmeal to cool slightly before serving. You can top it with more sliced nuts, fruit, honey, or your favorite paleo yogurt.

CHAPTER 3

Lunch Recipes

Quinoa with Chopped Fennel, Halved Grapes, Sliced Almonds, Thyme, Olive Oil, and Red Wine Vinegar.

(4 serves, 15 minutes preparation)

Ingredients:

- 1 cup washed quinoa.
- 1 bulb fennel, thinly sliced
- 1 cup red grapes, halved
- 1/4 cup slivered almonds.
- One tablespoon olive oil.
- 1 tablespoon of red wine vinegar.
- 1/2 teaspoon dried thyme.
- Add salt and pepper to taste.

Method:

- As directed on the package, prepare the quinoa.
- Meanwhile, place a skillet over medium heat with the olive oil. Cook until the fennel is tender, about 5 minutes.

- Add grapes and heat for another minute, or until warmed through.
- In a large bowl, combine the cooked quinoa, fennel, grapes, almonds, red wine vinegar, thyme, salt, and pepper. Toss to coat, and serve warm.

Bone Broth with Chicken and Brown Rice Noodles.

(2 serves, 20 minutes preparation, 30 minutes cooking)

Ingredients:

- Four cups of bone broth.
- One boneless, skinless chicken breast, cooked and shredded
- 1/2 cup brown rice noodles, cooked according to package directions.
- 1/2 cup chopped veggies (carrots, celery, and mushrooms).
- 1 tablespoon of chopped fresh parsley
- Add salt and pepper to taste.

Method:

- Heat bone broth in a saucepan over medium heat. Simmer for five minutes, or until the veggies are tender.

- Add shredded chicken and cooked brown rice noodles to the broth. Simmer for 5 minutes until heated thoroughly.

- Garnish with fresh parsley and season with salt and pepper as desired.

Paleo Meatballs with Zoodles

(4 serves, 20 minutes preparation, 20 minutes cooking)

Ingredients:

- One pound of ground meat (beef, lamb, turkey)
- One-half cup almond flour
- One-quarter cup chopped onion
- 1 egg
- One teaspoon of Italian seasoning
- Add salt and pepper to taste.
- Two zucchini spiralized into zoodles.

Method:

- 200°C, or 400°F, should be the oven temperature..
- In a bowl, combine the ground meat, almond flour, onion, egg, Italian seasoning, salt, and pepper. Mix thoroughly to create meatballs.

- Place the meatballs on a baking sheet and bake for 15-20 minutes, or until thoroughly cooked.

- Meanwhile, place a skillet over medium heat with the olive oil. Cook the zoodles for about 5 minutes, or until they are soft.

- Arrange meatballs on top of zoodles and enjoy.

Southwest Paleo Chicken with Fries

(2 serves, 20 minutes preparation, 20 minutes cooking)

Ingredients:

- Two boneless and skinless chicken breasts.

- One teaspoon of chili powder

- 1/2 teaspoon cumin.

- 1/4 teaspoon paprika.

- Add salt and pepper to taste.

- 2 thinly sliced sweet potatoes.

- One tablespoon olive oil.

- Avocado slices (optional).

- Chopped cilantro (optional).

Method:

- Chili powder, cumin, paprika, salt, and pepper are used to season the chicken breasts.
- 200°C, or 400°F, should be the oven temperature.. Toss sweet potato slices with olive oil and place on a baking sheet. Bake for 15 to 20 minutes, or until soft and crispy.
- While potatoes are baking, sauté chicken breasts in a pan over medium heat until done.
- Top the sweet potato fries with sliced chicken, avocado, and chopped cilantro (optional).

Cheesy Vegan Broccoli Soup

(4 serves, 15 minutes preparation, 20 minutes cooking)

Ingredients:

- One head of broccoli, chopped
- 1 onion, chopped
- 2 garlic cloves, minced
- Four cups of veggie broth.
- 1 can of coconut milk (13.5 oz)
- 1/2 cup of nutritional yeast.
- One teaspoon curry powder.
- Add salt and pepper to taste.

Method:

- Cook the onion and garlic in a saucepan over medium heat until tender.
- Bring broccoli and vegetable broth to a boil. After lowering the heat, simmer the broccoli for ten minutes, or until it becomes tender.
- Remove from heat and purée with an immersion blender or in batches in a conventional blender until smooth.
- Mix in the coconut milk, nutritional yeast, curry powder, salt, and pepper. Heat thoroughly without boiling.
- Optional garnish: nutritional yeast or chopped fresh herbs.

Chicken Pesto Stuffed Sweet Potatoes

(2 serves, 20 minutes preparation, 20 minutes cooking)

Ingredients:

- Two large sweet potatoes, cooked and half
- 1 or 2 boneless, skinless chicken breasts, cooked and shredded
- One-half cup pesto
- 1/4 cup crumbled feta cheese.
- Sun-dried tomatoes (optional).
- Chopped fresh basil (optional).

Method:

- 200°C, or 400°F, should be the oven temperature.. Bake sweet potatoes for approximately 40 minutes, or until cooked.
- While potatoes are baking, cook and shred chicken breasts.
- Mix together the shredded chicken, pesto, and feta cheese in a bowl.
- After cooking the potatoes, scrape off some of the flesh, leaving a boat-like shell. Fill the potato halves with the chicken pesto mixture.
- Garnish with sun-dried tomatoes and chopped basil (optional).
- Broil for a few minutes, until lightly browned and melted.

Chipotle Chicken Fajita Bowl.

(2 serves, 20 minutes preparation, 20 minutes cooking)

Ingredients:

- One boneless, skinless chicken breast, cut
- One teaspoon of chipotle powder
- 1/2 teaspoon cumin.
- 1/4 teaspoon of smoked paprika
- Add salt and pepper to taste.

- 1 bell pepper, sliced

- 1 onion, sliced

- One avocado, sliced

- One cup of cooked brown rice.

- Chopped cilantro (optional).

- Lime wedges (Optional)

Method:

- Season the chicken with chipotle powder, cumin, paprika, salt, and pepper.

- Cook the chicken in a skillet over medium heat until cooked through.

- Cook the bell pepper and onion in the same pan until softened.

- In bowls, combine cooked brown rice, chicken, bell pepper, onion, avocado slices, and chopped cilantro (optional), and lime wedges.

Asian Chicken Thighs with Spicy Green Beans

(4 serves, 20 minutes preparation, 20 minutes cooking)

Ingredients:

- 4 boneless and skinless chicken thighs.
- One tablespoon of soy sauce.
- One tablespoon of rice vinegar.
- 1 teaspoon honey.
- 1/2 tsp minced ginger.
- 1/4 teaspoon garlic powder.
- 1/4 teaspoon of red pepper flakes (optional)
- 1 pound trimmed green beans.
- Sesame seeds (optional).

Method:

- Mix together soy sauce, rice vinegar, honey, ginger, garlic powder, and red pepper flakes (optional). Marinate the chicken in the marinade for a minimum of 15 minutes.
- 200°C, or 400°F, should be the oven temperature.. Place the green beans on a baking pan and roast for 10 minutes.
- Place chicken thighs on top of green beans and bake for an additional 15-20 minutes, or until chicken is thoroughly cooked.
- Sprinkle with sesame seeds (optional) and serve.

Mediterranean Power Bowl

(2 serves, 15 minutes preparation, 10 minutes cooking)

Ingredients:

- 1 cup cooked quinoa.
- 1/2 cup of chopped veggies (tomatoes, cucumbers, bell peppers).
- 1/4 cup crumbled feta cheese.
- 1/4 cup sliced Kalamata olives.
- 1/4 cup hummus.
- One-quarter cup olive oil
- One tablespoon of lemon juice.
- Fresh oregano or parsley, chopped

Method:

- As directed on the package, prepare the quinoa.
- While the quinoa is cooking, chop the vegetables and prepare the remaining ingredients.
- In a mixing bowl, add cooked quinoa, veggies, feta cheese, olives, hummus, olive oil, lemon juice, and chopped parsley or oregano.
- Toss until coated and serve.

Salmon, Asparagus, and Wild Rice

(4 serves, 20 minutes preparation, 20 minutes cooking)

Ingredients:

- Four salmon fillets.
- One tablespoon olive oil.
- Add salt and pepper to taste.
- 1 bunch asparagus, trimmed
- 1 cup washed wild rice.
- Two cups of veggie broth.
- 1/4 cup minced parsley (optional).

Method:

- Preheat the oven to 400°F (200° C).
- Season the salmon fillets with olive oil, salt, and pepper on both sides.
- Place the asparagus on a baking sheet and toss with olive oil and salt. Spread into a single layer.
- Place salmon fillets on top of asparagus.
- Bake for 15-20 minutes, or until the salmon is thoroughly cooked and readily flaked.
- While the salmon and asparagus boil, prepare the wild rice in vegetable broth according to package directions.

- Once cooked, fluff the rice with a fork and add the chopped parsley (optional).
- Serve wild rice first, then fish and asparagus. Enjoy!

CHAPTER 4

Dinner Recipes

Ground Beef Stuffed Peppers

(4 serves, 20 minutes preparation, 30 minutes cooking)

Ingredients:

- Four bell peppers, halved and seeded
- One pound of ground beef
- 1/2 cup of diced onion.
- 1/2 cup chopped bell pepper (a different color than the halves)
- 1/4 cup of chopped mushrooms.
- Half cup cooked brown rice (optional)
- 1 can (14.5 oz) chopped tomatoes (undrained)
- One tablespoon of tomato paste.
- One teaspoon of chili powder
- 1/2 teaspoon cumin.
- Add salt and pepper to taste.

Method:

- 200°C, or 400°F, should be the oven temperature..
- Cook the onion, bell pepper, and mushrooms in a skillet over medium heat until softened.
- Add the ground beef and heat until browned, breaking it up with a spoon.
- Mix in the cooked brown rice (optional), diced tomatoes, tomato paste, chili powder, cumin, salt, and pepper. Simmer for 5 minutes until thick.
- Fill bell pepper halves with meat mixture. Place in a baking dish and bake for 20-25 minutes, or until peppers are soft and filling is thoroughly cooked.

Salmon with Roasted Vegetables

(4 serves, 20 minutes preparation, 20 minutes cooking)

Ingredients:

- Four salmon fillets.
- One tablespoon olive oil.
- Add salt and pepper to taste.
- 1 head of broccoli, chopped into florets
- 1/2 cup of chopped red onion.
- 1/4 cup of chopped red bell pepper.

- One tablespoon of lemon juice.

Method:

- 200°C, or 400°F, should be the oven temperature.. Line a baking sheet with parchment paper.
- Toss broccoli, red onion, and red bell pepper in olive oil and season with salt and pepper. Spread evenly on the prepared baking sheet.
- Season the salmon fillets with olive oil, salt, and pepper. Place on top of the vegetables.
- Roast for 15-20 minutes, or until the salmon is fully cooked and easily flaked, and the veggies are soft.
- Drizzle lemon juice over fish before serving (optional).

Chicken Stir-Fry

(4 servings, 15 minutes preparation, 20 minutes cooking)

Ingredients:

- 1 pound boneless and skinless chicken breasts, sliced
- One tablespoon of arrowroot powder.
- One teaspoon of coconut oil.
- 1/2 cup of chopped veggies (broccoli, carrots, bell peppers).
- One-quarter cup chopped onion

- One-quarter cup chicken broth
- One tablespoon of tamari or soy sauce.
- One tablespoon of rice vinegar.
- 1 teaspoon grated ginger.
- 1/2 teaspoon garlic powder.
- A pinch of red pepper flakes (optional).
- Sesame seeds (optional).

Method:

- Coat the chicken pieces in arrowroot powder.
- Cook coconut oil in a skillet or wok over medium-high heat. Cook the chicken until browned on all sides.
- Cook the veggies and onion for about 5 minutes, or until softened.
- In a small bowl, combine the chicken broth, tamari or soy sauce, rice vinegar, ginger, garlic powder, and red pepper flakes (optional).
- Stir in the sauce and cook for about 2 minutes, or until it thickens.
- Serve over cooked rice or zoodles, topped with sesame seeds (optional).

Tuna Salad Lettuce Wraps

(4 servings, 15-minute prep)

Ingredients:

- Two cans of tuna (12 oz each), drained and flakes
- 1/2 cup of chopped celery.
- 1/4 cup diced red onion
- 1/4 cup chopped apples
- 2 tablespoons mayonnaise.
- One tablespoon of lemon juice.
- 1/2 tsp Dijon mustard
- Add salt and pepper to taste.
- Four huge lettuce leaves.

Method:

- In a bowl, mix together the tuna, celery, red onion, apple, mayonnaise, lemon juice, Dijon mustard, salt, and pepper. Mix well.
- Wash and dry the lettuce leaves.
- Spoon the tuna salad mixture into each lettuce leaf and roll up to serve.

Steak with Chimichurri

(2 servings, 20 minutes preparation, 10 minutes cooking)

Ingredients:

- Two ribeye steaks.
- One tablespoon olive oil.
- Add salt and pepper to taste.

Chimichurri Sauce:

- 1/4 cup of chopped fresh parsley.
- 1/4 cup of chopped fresh cilantro.
- 2 garlic cloves, minced
- One-quarter cup olive oil
- 1 tablespoon of red wine vinegar.
- 1/2 teaspoon of dried oregano.
- Add salt and pepper to taste.

Method:

- Make the Chimichurri sauce: In a small mixing bowl, add chopped parsley, cilantro, garlic, olive oil, red wine vinegar, oregano, salt, and pepper. Stir thoroughly and let aside for at least 30 minutes to let the flavors combine.
- Cook the steak: Season the ribeye steaks well with salt and pepper. Heat a grill pan or cast iron skillet on medium-high

until extremely hot. Add the steaks and cook for 4-5 minutes per side for medium-rare, or until desired doneness.

- Rest and serve: Place the cooked steaks on a platter and allow them to rest for 5-10 minutes before slicing. This allows the liquids to redistribute throughout the meat, creating a more delicate texture.

- Assemble and serve: Once the steaks have rested, slice them and generously sprinkle with the prepared Chimichurri sauce. Serve the steak with grilled veggies, roasted potatoes, or a simple salad.

Shrimp Scampi

(4 serves, 20 minutes preparation, 15 minutes cooking)

Ingredients:

- 1 pound of big shrimp, peeled and deveined
- 2 tablespoons olive oil.
- 2 garlic cloves, minced
- 1/4 cup of dry white wine.
- One tablespoon of lemon juice.
- 1/4 cup of chopped fresh parsley.
- 1/4 teaspoon of dried oregano.
- Add salt and pepper to taste.

- One tablespoon butter (optional)

Method:

- Heat the olive oil in a large skillet over medium heat. Cook for about 30 seconds, or until the garlic becomes aromatic.
- Cook the shrimp until pink and opaque, about 2-3 minutes per side. Remove from the pan and set aside.
- In the pan, combine white wine, lemon juice, parsley, oregano, salt, and pepper. Bring to a simmer and cook for 1-2 minutes, or until slightly reduced.
- Stir in the butter (optional) until melted and smooth.
- Return the shrimp to the pan and toss to coat with the sauce.
- Serve immediately with cauliflower rice or zucchini noodles for a paleo-friendly alternative.

Poached Cod with Lemon and Dill

(4 serves, 15 minutes preparation, 15 minutes cooking)

Ingredients:

- Four cod fillets.
- Four cups of water.
- One-half cup white wine
- One-quarter cup lemon juice

- 1 tablespoon of chopped fresh dill

- 1/2 teaspoon salt.

- 1/4 teaspoon black peppercorns.

Method:

- In a large pot, heat the water, white wine, lemon juice, dill, salt, and peppercorns until simmering.

- Carefully place the fish fillets into the cooking liquid and cover the saucepan.

- Poach the cod for 7-8 minutes, or until opaque and fully cooked.

- Remove the fish from the pot and drain it on paper towels.

- Serve alongside roasted veggies or a simple salad.

Chicken Soup with Zoodles

(4 servings, 20 minutes preparation, 30 minutes cooking)

Ingredients:

- 1 pound of boneless, skinless chicken breasts or thighs, chopped

- One tablespoon olive oil.

- 1 onion, chopped

- two carrots, diced

- two celery stalks, chopped

- Four cups of chicken broth.

- One teaspoon dried thyme.

- 1/2 teaspoon salt.

- One-quarter teaspoon black pepper

- Two zucchini spiralized into zoodles.

Method:

- Heat the olive oil in a big pot over medium heat. Cook the onion, carrots, and celery for about 5 minutes, or until softened.

- Cook chicken until browned on all sides.

- Add chicken broth, thyme, salt, and pepper. Bring to a boil, then reduce the heat and simmer for 15 minutes.

- Cook for an additional 5 minutes, or until the zoodles are cooked but still somewhat al dente.

- If wanted, garnish with fresh parsley and serve warm.

Beef with Broccoli

(4 servings, 20 minutes preparation, 20 minutes cooking)

Ingredients:

- 1 pound flank steak, finely cut.
- One tablespoon of arrowroot powder.
- One teaspoon of coconut oil.
- 1 head of broccoli, chopped into florets
- One-half cup beef broth
- One tablespoon of tamari or soy sauce.
- One teaspoon of rice vinegar
- 1 teaspoon grated ginger.
- 1/2 teaspoon garlic powder.
- A pinch of red pepper flakes (optional).
- Sesame seeds (optional).

Method:

- Coat flank steak pieces in arrowroot powder.
- Cook coconut oil in a skillet or wok over medium-high heat. Cook steak until browned on all sides.
- Add broccoli and simmer until mushy, about 5 minutes.
- In a small bowl, whisk together beef broth, tamari or soy sauce, rice vinegar, ginger, garlic powder, and red pepper flakes (optional).

- Stir in the sauce and cook for about 2 minutes, or until it thickens.
- Serve over cooked rice or zoodles, topped with sesame seeds (optional).

Turkey Meatballs with Marinara Sauce

(4 serves, 20 mins prep, 20 mins cook)

Ingredients:

- 1 lb ground turkey
- 1/4 cup almond flour
- One-quarter cup chopped onion
- 1/4 cup chopped parsley
- 1 egg
- One teaspoon of Italian seasoning
- Add salt and pepper to taste.

Marinara sauce:

- 1 (28 oz) can crushed tomatoes
- One tablespoon olive oil.
- 1 clove garlic, minced
- 1/2 teaspoon of dried oregano.
- 1/4 tsp dried basil

- Add salt and pepper to taste.

Method:

- Prepare the meatballs: In a large bowl, combine ground turkey, almond flour, chopped onion, chopped parsley, egg, Italian seasoning, salt, and pepper. Mix thoroughly to produce a sticky mixture.
- Shape the meatballs: Roll the mixture into 1-inch balls.
- Cook the meatballs: You can bake, pan-fry, or put them in the crockpot. Here are three choices:
- Bake: Preheat the oven to 400°F (200°C). Line a baking sheet with parchment paper and arrange the meatballs on it. Bake for 15-20 minutes, or until thoroughly done.
- Skillet-fry: Heat the olive oil in a skillet over medium heat. Cook the meatballs until browned on all sides, about 5-7 minutes per side.
- Crockpot: In a slow cooker, combine the meatballs and your preferred marinara sauce recipe (see below). Cook on low for 4-6 hours, or until the meatballs are cooked through.
- Make marinara sauce (optional): If you don't want to use store-bought marinara, you may make it yourself following this simple recipe: In a medium saucepan, heat the olive oil. Cook for about 30 seconds, or until the garlic becomes aromatic. Combine smashed tomatoes, oregano, basil, salt,

and pepper. Bring to a simmer, then cook for 15 minutes, or until thickened.

- Serve: Remove any extra oil from the cooked meatballs. Serve hot with your preferred marinara sauce, zoodles, roasted veggies, or a side salad.

CHAPTER 5

Snack Recipes

Celery Sticks with Almond Butter

(2 servings, 5 minute prep)

Ingredients:

- Two celery stalks, chopped into sticks.
- One-quarter cup almond butter
- Optional: sprinkle with cinnamon.

Method:

- Wash and dry the celery sticks.
- Drizzle or dip celery sticks in almond butter.
- Add cinnamon for an added flavor boost (optional).

Apple Cinnamon Paleo Coffee Cake

(8 serves, 30 minutes preparation, 45 minutes cooking)

Ingredients:

- Two peeled and grated Granny Smith apples
- One-half cup almond flour
- One-quarter cup coconut flour

- 1/4 cup chopped walnuts.

- One-quarter teaspoon baking powder

- One-half teaspoon cinnamon

- 1/4 teaspoon nutmeg.

- One-quarter cup honey

- 1 egg

- 1 tablespoon melted coconut oil.

Method:

- Preheat the oven to 350°F (175° C). Grease a small baking dish (about 8x8 inches).

- In a large mixing bowl, add grated apples, almond flour, coconut flour, walnuts, baking powder, cinnamon, and nutmeg. Stir thoroughly.

- In a separate bowl, combine honey, egg, and melted coconut oil.

- Mix the wet components with the dry ingredients until just mixed.

- Pour the batter into the prepared baking dish and spread evenly.

- Bake for 45 to 50 minutes, or until golden brown and a toothpick inserted into the center comes out clean.

- Allow to cool somewhat before serving. Serve your paleo coffee cake warm or at room temperature.

Banana with Almond Butter

(2 serves, 2 minutes preparation)

Ingredients:

- One ripe banana.
- One-quarter cup almond butter

Method:

- Peel and slice the banana.
- Spread almond butter on banana slices or dip them into almond butter.

Beef Jerky with Dried Fruit

(1 serving, 2-minute preparation)

Ingredients:

- One ounce of beef jerky.
- 1/4 cup dried fruit (e.g. cranberries, raisins, or apricots).

Method:

- Combine beef jerky and dried fruit for a handy, protein-rich snack.

Hardboiled Eggs

(2 serves, 10 minutes preparation, 12 minutes cooking)

Ingredients:

- Two big eggs.

Method:

- Put eggs in a pot and cover with cold water. Bring water to a boil, then remove from heat and cover.
- Allow eggs to sit for 10–12 minutes.
- Drain the water and let the eggs cool under cold running water. Peel and enjoy.

Rice Cake with Sun Butter, Jam, or Fresh Strawberries

(1 serving, 2 minutes prep)

Ingredients:

- One gluten-free rice cake.
- 2 tablespoons sunflower butter
- One tablespoon jam or a handful of fresh strawberries.

Method:

- Spread sunflower butter on a rice cake.

- Garnish with jam or fresh strawberries.

Kale, Kimchi, and Breakfast Sausages

(1 serving, 5 minute prep)

Ingredients:

- 1 handful chopped kale.

- One tablespoon of kimchi

- Two cooked and sliced breakfast sausages.

Method:

- Mix chopped kale, kimchi, and cooked sausage slices in a bowl.

- Toss to coat, then enjoy.

Gluten-Free Oatmeal With Wild Blueberries And Honey

(1 serving, 5 minutes prep, 5 minutes cook)

Ingredients:

- 1/2 cup gluten-free oatmeal
- 1 cup water or unsweetened almond milk.
- 1/4 cup wild blueberries.
- One teaspoon of honey (optional)

Method:

- In a small saucepan, heat the water or almond milk until it simmers.
- Cook gluten-free oats for 5 minutes, stirring occasionally.
- Remove from heat and add wild blueberries and honey (optional).
- Enjoy warm.

Coconut Chips

(1 serving, 2 minutes preparation)

Ingredients:

- 1/4 cup unsweetened coconut chips.

Method:

- Enjoy a handful of unsweetened coconut chips for a naturally sweet and filling treat.

Brazil Nuts

(1 serving, 2 minutes preparation)

Ingredients:

- 3–4 Brazil nuts

Method:

- Enjoy a small handful of Brazil nuts as a nutrient-dense snack high in selenium and healthy fats.

CHAPTER 6

Dessert Recipes

Chocolate Avocado Mousse

(4 serves, 15-minute prep)

Ingredients:

- Two ripe avocados, peeled and pitted.
- 1/3 cup unsweetened cocoa powder.
- 1/4 cup honey or maple syrup.
- One-quarter cup coconut milk
- 1/2 teaspoon of vanilla extract.
- A pinch of sea salt.

Method:

- Using a high-powered blender, combine all ingredients until smooth and creamy.
- Divide among serving cups and chill for at least 30 minutes for optimal texture.
- Add your favourite paleo-friendly toppings, such as fresh berries, chopped almonds, or coconut flakes (optional).

Baked Apples with Nuts and Spices

(4 serves, 20 minutes preparation, 40 minutes cooking)

Ingredients:

- Four apples, cored and halved
- 1/4 cup chopped pecans or walnuts.
- 1/4 cup raisins, chopped dates
- One-quarter teaspoon cinnamon
- 1/4 teaspoon nutmeg.
- A pinch of ginger (optional).
- One tablespoon butter or ghee (optional)

Method:

- Preheat the oven to 375° F (190° C).
- In a bowl, combine chopped nuts, raisins, spices, and butter (optional).
- Fill the apple halves with the filling mixture.
- Place the apples in a baking dish, sliced side up.
- Bake for 40 to 45 minutes, or until the apples are soft and the filling is golden brown.
- Serve warm with more chopped nuts or a dab of honey (optional).

Coconut Milk Popsicles

(4-6 servings, 15-minute prep, 4-hour freeze).

Ingredients:

- 1 can (13.5 oz) of full-fat coconut milk
- 1/4 cup honey or maple syrup.
- 1/2 teaspoon of vanilla extract.
- A pinch of sea salt.

Method:

- Combine all of the ingredients and blend until smooth.
- Pour into Popsicle molds or small paper cups.
- Freeze for a minimum of 4 hours, or until solid.
- Enjoy as a cool and creamy paleo treat.

Fruit Salad with Coconut Whipped Cream

(4 serves, 15-minute prep)

Ingredients:

• Two cups mixed berries (strawberries, blueberries, raspberries)

• One cup of diced mango or pineapple

• 1/2 cup unsweetened coconut cream.

• 1/4 teaspoon of vanilla extract.

• A pinch of sea salt.

Method:

• Whip coconut cream, vanilla extract, and sea salt until soft peaks form (do not over whip).

• Mix the diced fruits in a bowl.

• Garnish with coconut whipped cream and enjoy.

Paleo Brownies

(8 servings, 20 minutes preparation, 25 minutes cooking)

Ingredients:

- One-half cup almond flour
- One-quarter cup coconut flour
- 1/4 cup cocoa powder.
- 1/4 cup honey or maple syrup.
- 1/4 cup melted coconut oil.
- 1 egg
- One-half teaspoon baking powder
- A pinch of sea salt.

Method:

- Preheat the oven to 350°F (175° C). Line an 8-by-8-inch baking pan with parchment paper.
- In a bowl, combine the dry ingredients (almond flour, coconut flour, cocoa powder, baking powder, and salt).
- In a separate bowl, whisk together the wet ingredients (honey, coconut oil, egg).
- Combine wet and dry ingredients, stirring until just combined.
- Pour the batter into the prepared pan and distribute evenly.
- Bake for 25-30 minutes, or until a toothpick inserted into the center yields moist crumbs.
- Cool completely before cutting and serving.

Almond Flour Pancakes with Berries

(2 servings, 15 minutes preparation, 10 minutes cooking)

Ingredients:

- One-quarter cup almond flour
- One-quarter cup coconut flour
- One-quarter teaspoon baking powder
- A pinch of sea salt.
- 1 egg

- 1/4 cup of unsweetened almond milk.

- 1/4 teaspoon of vanilla extract.

- Coconut oil for greasing the pan.

- Fresh berries (for topping)

- Honey, maple syrup (optional)

Method:

- Combine the dry ingredients (almond flour, coconut flour, baking powder, and salt) in a mixing bowl.

- In a separate bowl, combine the wet ingredients (egg, almond milk, and vanilla essence).

- Combine wet and dry ingredients, stirring until just combined. Don't over mix the pancakes, as this will make them tough.

- Cook in a lightly oiled pan over medium heat.

- Pour the batter onto the pan in 1/4 cup parts, making little pancakes.

- Cook for 2-3 minutes on each side, or until golden brown and cooked through.

- Optional toppings include fresh berries, whipped cream, and a drizzle of honey or maple syrup.

Roasted Figs with Honey and Walnuts

(4 serves, 15 minutes preparation, 20 minutes cooking)

Ingredients:

- Four ripe figs, quartered
- One spoonful of honey.
- 1/4 cup chopped walnuts.
- A pinch of cinnamon.
- A pinch of sea salt.

Method:

- 200°C, or 400°F, should be the oven temperature.. Line a baking sheet with parchment paper.
- Toss the fig quarters with honey, walnuts, cinnamon, and salt.
- Spread out on the prepared baking sheet and roast for 20-25 minutes, or until the figs are somewhat softened and caramelized.
- Serve warm or room temperature.

Chia Seed Pudding with Fruit and Nuts

(4 serves, 15-minute prep, 4-hour chill)

Ingredients:

- 1/4 cup of chia seeds.
- One cup unsweetened almond milk.
- 1/4 cup honey or maple syrup.
- 1/2 teaspoon of vanilla extract.
- A pinch of sea salt.
- 1 cup mixed berries (strawberries, raspberries, blueberries)
- 1/4 cup chopped pecans or almonds.

Method:

- In a dish, combine the chia seeds, almond milk, honey, vanilla essence, and salt. Stir thoroughly and allow it sit for 5 minutes, or until the mixture thickens.
- Cover and refrigerate for at least 4 hours, preferably overnight for optimal results.
- When ready to serve, divide the pudding into bowls. Garnish with fresh berries and chopped nuts.

Baked Sweet Potato with Cinnamon and Nuts

(2 serves, 15 minutes preparation, 45 minutes cooking)

Ingredients:

- Scrub two medium sweet potatoes and pierce with a fork.
- One tablespoon of olive oil.
- One-half teaspoon cinnamon
- A pinch of sea salt.
- 1/4 cup chopped walnuts or pecans (optional).

Method:

- 200°C, or 400°F, should be the oven temperature..
- Rub sweet potatoes with olive oil and season with cinnamon and salt.
- Place on a baking pan and bake for 45-50 minutes, or until fork-tender.
- Cut open and serve with chopped nuts (optional).

Dark Chocolate with Berries

(4 serves, 2 mins prep)

Ingredients:

- 1 ounce dark chocolate (70% or higher cacao content)
- 1/2 cup mixed berries (strawberries, blueberries, raspberries)

Method:

- Break dark chocolate into squares.
- Dip berries in dark chocolate or melt chocolate and drizzle over berries.
- Enjoy this simple and tasty paleo-friendly dessert.

CONCLUSION

As we reach the final chapter of the Hashimoto Paleo Cookbook, our hearts swell with appreciation for your company on this transforming voyage. Your devotion to studying the pages of thyroid-friendly recipes and embracing the Hashimoto's Paleo Lifestyle is a testimonial to your dedication to well-being.

In parting, we encourage you to carry forward the flame of the Hashimoto's Paleo Lifestyle with steadfast commitment. Each meal is a simple but profound act of self-love, contributing to the tapestry of your well-being. Consistency is the key, and your journey towards vitality is a marathon, not a sprint. May the delicacies you've discovered within these pages continue to influence your daily choices.

As you travel this route, we emphasize the critical role of healthcare experts in your specific journey. Their counsel ensures that your choices correspond neatly with your unique health demands. Your interaction with medical specialists adds to a complete and tailored approach to Hashimoto's care.

Lastly, we invite you to share your ideas with us. Drop a positive feedback about your experience with the Hashimoto Paleo Cookbook. Your insights are vital, helping us grow and motivating others to begin on their own journeys.

May your days be filled with wholesome meals, rejuvenated energy, and the delight that comes from embracing a lifestyle that appreciates the remarkable synergy of health and flavour.

With Heartfelt Thanks,

Christiana White

2-Week Meal Plan

Week 1

Monday

• Breakfast: Keto Breakfast Burger with Avocado Buns

• Lunch: Quinoa with chopped fennel, halved grapes, slivered almonds, thyme, olive oil, and red wine vinegar

• Dinner: Ground Beef Stuffed Peppers

• Snacks: Celery Sticks with Almond Butter, Apple cinnamon paleo coffee cake

• Dessert: Chocolate Avocado Mousse

Tuesday

• Breakfast: Paleo Freezer Breakfast Burritos

• Lunch: Bone broth with chicken and brown rice noodles

• Dinner: Salmon with Roasted Vegetables

• Snacks: Banana with almond butter, Beef jerky and dried fruit

• Dessert: Baked Apples with Nuts and Spices

Wednesday

• Breakfast: Paleo Red Flannel Hash

• Lunch: Paleo meatballs with zoodles

• Dinner: Chicken Stir-Fry

• Snacks: Hardboiled eggs, Rice cake with sun butter and jam or fresh strawberries

• Dessert: Coconut Milk Popsicles

Thursday

• Breakfast: Keto Blueberry Muffins

• Lunch: Southwest paleo chicken and fries

• Dinner: Tuna Salad Lettuce Wraps

• Snacks: Kale, kimchi, and breakfast sausages, Coconut Chips

• Dessert: Fruit Salad with Coconut Whipped Cream

Friday

• Breakfast: Bacon and Egg Sweet Potato Pancake Breakfast Sandwich

• Lunch: Cheesy vegan broccoli soup

• Dinner: Steak with Chimichurri

• Snacks: Brazil nuts, Gluten free oats with wild blueberries and honey

• Dessert: Paleo Brownies

Saturday

• Breakfast: Loaded Paleo Breakfast Hash

• Lunch: Chicken pesto stuffed sweet potatoes

• Dinner: Shrimp Scampi

• Snacks: Celery Sticks with Almond Butter, Apple cinnamon paleo coffee cake

• Dessert: Almond Flour Pancakes with Berries

Sunday

- Breakfast: Make-Ahead Breakfast Sandwich
- Lunch: Chipotle chicken fajita bowl
- Dinner: Poached Cod with Lemon and Dill
- Snacks: Banana with almond butter, Beef jerky and dried fruit
- Dessert: Roasted Figs with Honey and Walnuts

Week 2

Monday

- Breakfast: Paleo Porridge with Caramelized Bananas
- Lunch: Asian chicken thighs and spicy green beans
- Dinner: Chicken Soup with Zoodles
- Snacks: Hardboiled eggs, Rice cake with sun butter and jam or fresh strawberries
- Dessert: Chia Seed Pudding with Fruit and Nuts

Tuesday

- Breakfast: Zucchini Carrot Muffins
- Lunch: Mediterranean power bowl
- Dinner: Beef and Broccoli
- Snacks: Kale, kimchi, and breakfast sausages, Coconut Chips
- Dessert: Baked Sweet Potato with Cinnamon and Nuts

Wednesday

• Breakfast: Baked Almond Quinoa and Oatmeal

• Lunch: Salmon, asparagus, and wild rice

• Dinner: Turkey Meatballs with Marinara Sauce

• Snacks: Brazil nuts, Gluten free oats with wild blueberries and honey

• Dessert: Dark Chocolate with Berries

Thursday

• Breakfast: Keto Breakfast Burger with Avocado Buns

• Lunch: Quinoa with chopped fennel, halved grapes, slivered almonds, thyme, olive oil, and red wine vinegar

• Dinner: Ground Beef Stuffed Peppers

• Snacks: Celery Sticks with Almond Butter, Apple cinnamon paleo coffee cake

• Dessert: Chocolate Avocado Mousse

Friday

• Breakfast: Paleo Freezer Breakfast Burritos

• Lunch: Bone broth with chicken and brown rice noodles

• Dinner: Salmon with Roasted Vegetables

• Snacks: Banana with almond butter, Beef jerky and dried fruit

• Dessert: Baked Apples with Nuts and Spices

Saturday

• Breakfast: Paleo Red Flannel Hash

• Lunch: Paleo meatballs with zoodles

• Dinner: Chicken Stir-Fry

• Snacks: Hardboiled eggs, Rice cake with sun butter and jam or fresh strawberries

• Dessert: Coconut Milk Popsicles

Sunday

• Breakfast: Keto Blueberry Muffins

• Lunch: Southwest paleo chicken and fries

• Dinner: Tuna Salad Lettuce Wraps

• Snacks: Kale, kimchi, and breakfast sausages, Coconut Chips

• Dessert: Fruit Salad with Coconut Whipped Cream

www.ingramcontent.com/pod-product-compliance
Lightning Source LLC
Chambersburg PA
CBHW050845260726
48660CB00006B/2455